Intermittent Fasting For Women

Eat What You Want and Still Lose Weight

By Kelly Fung and Catherine Fung

Table of Contents

Introduction

Did the title of the book surprise you? Wouldn't it be nice if you could eat what you want to eat and still lose weight? Not just that, doesn't it sound wonderful that you can lose weight without following a crash diet, expensive diet plans or have to count calories?

If that sounds good to you, then intermittent fasting may be the best diet for you!

Most of us tend to fast unknowingly. It is true! Your body fasts when you sleep, and you fast in between your meals. Intermittent fasting is a mere extension of this fasting period. It's easier than you think!

If you are a woman who is struggling with weight issues and you want to start this diet but you don't know where to begin, then this is the perfect book for you. You can achieve your health and weight loss goals without spending money on a gym membership or a fancy diet plan. In this book, you will learn about intermittent fasting and its effect on women, the different types of fasts, benefits and how you can lose weight while on a budget.

It's easier than you may think!

Chapter One:
Intermittent Fasting

Intermittent fasting is a system of dieting where you fast from between 12 to 16 hours or more a day. During your fasting period, you cannot take in any calories (barring a few exceptions, which are explained in detail in the subsequent chapters). While it may sound a little tricky to achieve, you may already be fasting without being aware of it. For instance, if you have your dinner at 8 p.m. and then the next meal you have is your breakfast the following day at 10 a.m., then you are in effect fasting for 14 hours! Yes, you are fasting, and you didn't even know that you were fasting.

Intermittent fasting may sound slightly technical. However, you are probably already unknowingly fasting. Before you learn what intermittent fasting is about, you should know the difference between fasting and fed states. After you eat, your body is in a fed state. In the fed state, your body will digest, absorb and assimilate nutrients from the food you have consumed. The main priority of your body in this state should be to burn fat. Most of us tend to stay in a fed state throughout the day, except when we sleep.

Intermittent fasting is beneficial because it helps your body enter a fasted state. In a "fasted" state, your body burns fat in order to provide energy. So, what is an intermittent fast? It merely means that you should fast for anywhere between 12 to

48 hours. The length of the fast is known as the fasting window. Your eating windows are the times that you eat.

Intermittent fasting oscillates between fasting and eating. During your fasting window, you can consume liquids without any or very few calories, like water, herbal tea, or even some broth. It is better to avoid calories when you fast, but you can include a couple of low calorie green vegetable juices to help maintain the nutrient requirements of your body. There are no hard and fast rules when it comes to intermittent fasting, and it is pretty subjective.

If you fast for less than 24 hours, you will have an eating window. The eating window is the time within which you can eat before the next fast starts. All of those who practice intermittent fasting limit their eating window to between 6 - 12 hours. The most common times for intermittent fasting are 12, 14, 16, and 18 hours. For instance, when you fast for 12 hours, your eating window will be 12 hours. You can start your eating window at 8 am in the morning and end it at 8 pm at night and then you can break your fast on the next day at 8 am.

Intermittent fasting offers women sustainable weight loss, increase in lean muscle, better energy, better response to cell stress, reduction in inflammation, oxidative stress and improved insulin sensitivity. It also triggers the production of growth hormone. You will learn more about these benefits in the coming chapters.

Intermittent fasting is popularly known as IF, and it is an excellent method to become lean and lose weight. It helps improve your energy levels, stamina, and cognitive functions.

Intermittent fasting is a great plan, and offers plenty of health benefits. However, the effects of intermittent fasting are dependent upon your biology. The effect that IF has on men is different than how a female body will experience it. A woman's body is usually sensitive to signs of starvation, and therefore it works differently, and often better for women. Finally, us women get a break!

Fasting and hormones

Intermittent fasting can cause a hormonal imbalance if you don't do it correctly. Women are naturally more sensitive to the signals of starvation. So, whenever your body feels that you are under-eating, it misinterprets it as starvation and increases the production of leptin and ghrelin. When this happens, you will feel hungry. Technically, your body doesn't need more food, but hormones tell you otherwise. Whenever a woman's body senses that it is heading toward starvation (regardless of whether it is intentional or not), it increases the production of hunger hormones. The two hormones that regulate hunger and give the body signals to eat are ghrelin and leptin. So, when there is an increase in the production of these hormones, you will feel hungry.

If there isn't sufficient food to survive, your body will shut down its reproductive system. The body won't procreate when it feels that it doesn't have sufficient nourishment to sustain itself and a fetus. It is the body's natural defense mechanism to prevent a potential pregnancy. The body will try to protect itself from pregnancy, even if you want to conceive. Your body cannot tell the difference between a fast that is self-imposed and starvation. It doesn't know the difference between starvation and intermittent fasting. Therefore, the default protective mechanism kicks in.

There are a couple of side effects of intermittent fasting that can cause hormonal imbalances. These imbalances can lead to irregular menstruation, amenorrhea in extreme cases, metabolic stress, the shrinking of ovaries, anxiety, depression, lack of sleep, and fertility issues.

All of the hormones in the body are interconnected, so when there is a shift in the equilibrium of one hormone, it affects the other hormones. Think of it as a domino effect. Hormones are messengers that control all of the bodily functions, from the production of energy, to digestion, metabolism and even the regulation of blood pressure. You don't want to disrupt the natural rhythm of these functions, do you? Because of all these drawbacks, you might wonder if you can still practice intermittent fasting. Well, don't let these side effects scare you. You can practice intermittent fasting safely, if you opt for a relaxed approach. When you don't extend your fast for too long, you can attain your health and weight loss goals quickly. You can also do this without interfering with your hormones in a negative way.

Most women try to ignore these hunger pangs, and it causes the signals to grow louder. Or worse, they try to ignore these cues and fail, and eventually begin to binge eat. Then many women try to balance it out by under-eating, and the cycle continues. This vicious cycle can throw your hormonal balance out of whack!

An animal study conducted on female rats in 2013 showed that fasting for excess periods of time led to a disruption in the menstrual cycle and ovaries shrank. The male rats experienced insomnia and a reduction in the production of testosterone. However, there are only a few human studies about the effects of intermittent fasting on men and women. Most of the data is based on animal studies. One thing that the studies agree on is that fasting for extremely long periods can at times lead to a hormonal imbalance in women. Well, it doesn't mean that intermittent fasting is terrible. No worries - there is a solution to this!

In the grand scheme of things, experimenting with IF is quite simple. For a woman, this small experiment can have a huge impact. Hormones are essential to regulate different functions in the body like ovulation. Ovulation is sensitive to the levels of energy present in the body. Think of the HPG axis (hypothalamic-pituitary-gonadal) as the air traffic controller in the human body. The hypothalamus secretes gonadotropin that releases the GnRH hormone. It, in turn, signals the pituitary gland to release a luteinizing hormone or LH and FSH (follicular stimulating hormone). These LH and FSH hormones act as the gonads or in simpler terms they are known as testes or ovaries.

In women, it triggers the secretion of estrogen and progesterone that are necessary to start ovulation and sustain pregnancy. On the other hand, it triggers the flow of testosterone and sperm in men. It is essential to time any GnRH pulses in the body. If it isn't timed correctly, it can throw the female cycle out of order. Not just that, GnRH pulses are also sensitive to different environmental factors and can be thrown off course by fasting.

The next question that we should address is "Why does IF affects female hormones differently than male hormones?" To be honest, no one has a solid answer to this question. Studies suggest that it could be due to kisspeptin (a molecule that resembles a protein that helps the neurons to communicate with one another). Kisspeptin helps to stimulate the production of GnRH in both men and women. It is also sensitive to other hormones like leptin, insulin and ghrelin that help to regulate hunger and satiety in the body. It is an interesting point to note that female mammals tend to have more kisspeptin in their system than the male ones. The higher the number of kisspeptin neurons, the higher the body's sensitivity to any changes in energy levels. This is a good reason why a woman shouldn't fast for prolonged periods of time and should instead take a gradual approach. However, let me remind you once again that all f this information is based on studies done on animals and not on humans.

Women consume less protein than men. Naturally, during a fast, a woman will consumes even less protein than usual. Lower intake of protein means a reduction in the level of amino acids. Amino acids are necessary to stimulate the estrogen receptors and also for the synthesis IGF-1 (it is an insulin-like growth factor) that the liver secretes. IGF-1 helps to thicken the uterine wall and helps with the reproductive cycle. Therefore, a diet that is low in protein can reduce fertility. It is important to understand that estrogen is necessary, not just for reproduction, but that estrogen receptors are present throughout a woman's body. They are present in the brain, GI tract, and even the bones. Therefore, a change in the level of estrogen can lead to a change in the overall metabolic function of the body.

Estrogen can affect cognitive abilities, mood, digestion, cell recovery, bone formation, and protein turnover. Estrogen regulates appetite and your energy balance. Estrogen modifies the peptides in the brainstem that signal when you feel full or hungry. It stimulates the neurons in the hypothalamus that regulate the production of hunger-regulating peptides. If there is a drop in estrogen, it can make you feel extremely hungry, and you will end up eating more than you usually do. Therefore, it is safe to say that estrogens are an essential metabolic regulator. Yes, estrogens are plural. The ratios of different estrogenic metabolites like estriol, estradiol and estrone tend to change over time. Before you hit menopause, the primary player is estradiol. After menopause, it's level drops and the concentration of estrone stay the same. The role of these estrogens is not yet entirely clear. However, as a general theory, it is said that a drop in the levels of estradiol can lead to an increase in the storage of fat in the body because fats are necessary to synthesize estradiol. It might also explain why a lot of women find it difficult to shed weight after menopause.

It doesn't sound fair, does it? Men can strut around looking ripped, and you might still struggle to see the outline of your leg muscles or abs. From an evolutionary perspective, you probably shouldn't try too hard to gain washboard abs. A diet that reduces your energy levels will certainly mess with your reproductive health. There is an intricate interdependency between the female body's link in fertility and energy levels. Again, from an evolutionary perspective, it does make sense.

In the mammalian world, human females are somewhat unique. Almost all mammals can terminate or even pause their pregnancy in unfavorable circumstances. Well, women cannot do so. In a woman, the maternal blood vessels are breached by the placenta, and therefore it puts the fetus in control. When the fetus needs more glucose, then it can easily restrict the production of insulin in the mother's body. The fetus can also cause the blood vessels of the mother to expand to increase the nutrients it needs. So, during pregnancy, the baby is in complete control and not the mother. This relationship that exists in the body at the time of pregnancy is known as a "maternal-fetal conflict." A mother cannot stop the growth of the fetus. Therefore, pregnancy at the wrong time, like during a famine, can be quite fatal. It is no wonder that the reproductive pathways in women are very sensitive to metabolic cues. However, you might wonder how does the body "know" this?

The hormonal balance in a woman is very sensitive to when, what, and how much we eat. How does the body determine scarcity of food? This goes back to all the evolution of the human body. If the levels of reserve fat go below a certain percentage, it will mess with the hormones and your menstrual cycle will become irregular or it might even stop. When you think about it, it does make sense. When you reduce your food intake, your body will use its fats to provide energy. Therefore, it is imperative that there is a proper energy balance in a woman's body to avoid any of the hormonal imbalances discussed above. It is not just the food you eat that matters. A negative balance of energy can result when you eat very little, when the food isn't nutritious, too much exercise, high stress, illnesses and little rest. A combination of any of these stressors can cause a negative energy balance in your body.

Yes, stress can be lead to negative energy levels in the body. Even a psychological stressor is as bad as a physical one. Our body cannot differentiate between a real and an imaginary threat (like stress or worry). Mental stress can lead to a change in hormonal balance in the body. Cortisol is the stress hormone, and it inhibits GnRH, and it can suppress the production of estrogen and progesterone. When stressed, progesterone is converted into cortisol, and increases the overall stress you experience. So, it worsens the condition. Even if your fat percentage is around 30, too much stress leads to an imbalance in your energy levels and it can disrupt your reproductive cycle. At least, this stands correct in theory.

So, what can you do now? Based on all that we know, intermittent fasting can have a slight effect on your reproductive health if you don't do it correctly. If you do want to opt for intermittent fasting, you should opt for a balanced approach and nothing that's too drastic. If you're going to try IF, you should keep certain things in mind. If you experience any of the following things, you should stop IF.

- If there are any irregularities in your menstrual cycle or any problems with your sleep or you experience lack of sleep.

- If you notice any hair fall, dry skin or acne.

- If you are always tired and you cannot recover from workouts easily.

- Your body is slow to heal.

- A reduction in your tolerance for stress or extreme mood swings.

- A decrease in your sex drive, extremely slow digestion, or when you always feel cold.

If you experience any of these symptoms, you should stop IF.

Anyone who doesn't fall under the following categories can follow intermittent fasting. If you are pregnant, have an eating disorder or are recovering from an eating disorder, experience chronic depression, under extreme stress or suffer from insomnia, you may want to consider fasting at a later time.

The energy needs of a pregnant woman are more than that of an ordinary woman and, therefore, you shouldn't fast if you want to start a family soon. If you think you are under chronic stress, or if you cannot sleep properly, it may be time to nurture your body and not put it under further stress. Also, if you struggle with an eating disorder or struggle with an eating disorder in the past, a diet that prescribes fasting may prove counterproductive. The best thing that you can do is learn about nutrition and listen to your body. Your body knows what it needs, and you must listen to it.

Chapter Two:
Benefits of Intermittent Fasting

Intermittent Fasting when there is an oscillation between periods of eating and fasting. There are several benefits offered by this diet and there are scientific studies as well as research that support these claims. In this section, we will cover the different benefits this diet offers.

Change in Cell Function

When you fast for a while, different changes take place in your body. For instance, your body will start a process of cellular repair and there will be changes in your hormone level. A difference in these levels makes it easier for the body to access the stored fat. You will notice that there is a reduction in the level of insulin and it helps increase the body's ability to burn fat. An increase in the human growth hormone helps to increase lean muscle and burn more fat than usual. Not just that, it also kick starts the process of cellular repair. Damaged cells are processed and other processes of cellular repair kick in. In addition, several changes take place within the genes and molecules that protect you against disease.

Weight Loss

The most obvious benefit of this diet is weight loss. When you follow intermittent fasting, the number of meals you eat will be reduced. When you eat less, the calories you consume will decrease as well. When the levels of insulin decline, growth hormone increases along with an increase in norepinephrine, which helps the body break down stored fat to provide energy. There is an increase in your metabolic rate when you fast, which helps the body burn more calories. The effect of intermittent fasting is two-fold. On the one hand, it increases your metabolic rate and therefore makes your body more efficient while burning fats. The reduction in the level of food you consume reduces your overall calorie intake. Both these conditions promote weight and fat loss. Also, most of the fats that your body burns come from the abdominal area. The fat in the abdominal region happens to be the most stubborn of all, which is why this diet is perfect for belly flab.

Lower the Risk of Diabetes

The most common health problem that plagues humanity these days, apart from obesity, is diabetes. High blood sugar leads to insulin resistance in the body. Intermittent fasting helps to reduce blood sugar and therefore helps reduce insulin resistance in the body . When your body becomes resistant to insulin, it leads to an increase in the blood sugar level and the vicious cycle goes on and on. If you opt for this diet, you can successfully reverse this condition.

Reduces Inflammation

Oxidative stress is one of the main reasons for inflammation in the body. Inflammation is the body's natural reaction to illness. However, excess inflammation is a painful condition and causes a host of diseases like arthritis. When the unstable molecules in the body, known as free radicals, react with other essential molecules like proteins and DNA, it causes inflammation. Intermittent fasting helps reduce inflammation and also offers protection against aging. Premature aging isn't desirable, now is it?

Heart's Health

Heart disease is the most significant killer in the world. Several risk factors increase the chance of heart disease. Intermittent fasting helps reduce risk factors like blood pressure, high cholesterol, inflammatory markers, blood sugar and blood triglycerides. When you can control these risk factors, you reduce the chance of suffering from cardiovascular disease. However, once again, a lot of research in this field is based on animal studies.

Cellular Repair

Autophagy is the process of waste removal in the body, and intermittent fasting helps to kick-start this process. The body breaks down and metabolizes broken, as well as dysfunctional, proteins. An increase in autophagy protects you from several degenerative diseases like cancer and Alzheimer's.

All these benefits help to increase your lifespan and help you lead a healthier life. Not only will you lose weight, but you can also improve your overall health just by following the intermittent fasting method.

Chapter Three: Methods of Fasting

There are different variations of intermittent fasting and in this section, you will learn about the best methods of intermittent fasting for women.

Crescendo Fasting

Intermittent Fasting is a simple fasting protocol, but it can be slightly hard on your body if you are new to it or if you jump in too quickly. So, listen up ladies, if you are new to intermittent fasting, then the best method of fasting is crescendo fasting. In this method of fasting, you need to fast for a couple of days a week instead of daily. It is the best form of intermittent fasting and is a gentle approach that will enable your body to get used to fasting gradually. A radical approach will not help your body; you'll need to start slowly. You can obtain all the benefits of intermittent fasting without causing any harmful hormonal imbalances.

When you properly follow the protocols of this diet, you can shed all the excess pounds you want . The rules of this fast are quite simple. You should fast for two or three days in a week and make sure that you don't fast on any consecutive days. For instance, you can fast on Tuesday, Thursday and Saturday. On the days you fast, keep your exercise protocol light. You can do basic cardio or light yoga. Make sure that your fasting period doesn't exceed 12-16 hours. On the days when you don't fast and you want to take up high-intensity exercises, you'll likely want to eat in order to maintain your energy levels.

Always keep your body hydrated. You can even have calorie-free beverages on your fasting days. If you decide to fast for two days a week, after two weeks you can add another day to it. However, you shouldn't exceed three days in a week and the fasting days should never be consecutive. If you want to, you can have about 5-8 grams of branched-chain amino acids (BCAAs) on the days you fast. BCAA's will help provide additional energy on the days you fast and also help to reduce hunger pangs and fatigue.

16/8 Method

This method is also popularly known as the Leangains method. It is a short routine of intermittent fasting that will help you burn body fat and improve your lean muscle. In this diet, you should fast for 16 hours daily, and your eating window is restricted to 8 hours a day. For instance, you can start your fast at 7 p.m. and then fast until 11 a.m. the following day. So, you can break your fast with a meal at noon and end with a meal at night before 7 p.m. If you start your fast on Monday night, it will extend until noon on Tuesday and so on. You can move onto this method of fasting after your body gets used to the previous method of fasting. This variant of intermittent fasting is quite simple. It can be as simple as skipping your breakfast instead of having your first meal at noon.

Most of us tend to lead busy lives, and hardly any of us have the time to eat breakfast. Yes, it is as simple as that. Skip your breakfast, have a nutritious lunch, a snack, and end your day with a nutritious dinner. You shouldn't have any snacks post dinner and no more late-night snacks. It will also help regulate your circadian rhythm. If you have dinner at 7 or 8 at night, you can give your body sufficient time to digest the meal before you go to bed.

24-Hour Protocol

Also known as the Eat-Stop-Eat diet. As the name suggests, in this variation of intermittent fasting, you should fast for 24 hours at a stretch. However, you shouldn't fast more than twice a week. You can start with one day and then increase it to two days a week. As mentioned, you should never fast on two consecutive days. You can select your fasting window, and you should stick to it. You can start your fast at 8 p.m. and end it on 8 p.m. on the following day. You can fast on Monday and Wednesday. You'll need to fast for 24 hours in a day. Therefore, you will not have an eating window during this fast. While you fast, you can have plenty of calorie-free beverages. So you can have your coffee, but don't add any sugar, cream or milk to it. Herbal teas and water should be your go-to drinks. If you want, you can even spruce up your regular drinking water by adding a couple of slices of lemon and sprigs of mint.

5:2 Diet

The 5:2 diet is also known as the Fast Diet and on this diet, you should fast for two days a week. You might wonder what the difference is between this diet and the crescendo method. Unlike the crescendo method, on the days you fast, you shouldn't exceed 500 calories. In the crescendo method, you are free to eat anything you want after your fasting window ends. However, in this method, you can eat throughout the day, but you have a calorie restriction to follow. So, you will have to consume 500 calories twice a week and eat properly on the other days. You fast for two days and eat as usual on the other days of the week. You shouldn't fast on consecutive days. If you want, you can have one meal of 500 calories while you fast or break it up into smaller meals. It is a safe method of dieting.

There are a couple of general rules that you should keep in mind when you decide to follow any of the intermittent fasting protocols. You shouldn't fast for more than 24 hours at any given point in time. An ideal fast can last between 12 to 16 hours and nothing beyond it. Never fast on consecutive days. During the initial days of fasting, you shouldn't fast for more than two or three days, even if the fasting window doesn't exceed 16 hours on a fasting day. Keep your exercise schedule light on the fasting days and be sure to stay thoroughly hydrated.

Chapter Four:
Weight Loss on a Budget

Intermittent fasting does sound like a proper diet, doesn't it? Well, let me sweeten the deal further. You can lose weight while you stay on a budget. Now, that does sound infinitely better, doesn't it? This applies especially in today's world where different fad diets burn a hole in your pocket. In this section, you will learn tips that you can follow to shed excess pounds while on a budget.

Water, water, and more water

It is quintessential that you keep your body thoroughly hydrated while you follow a diet. Water helps to hydrate your body, clear your skin, flush out toxins and even fill you up. Regardless of the intermittent fasting protocol that you want to follow, you should have plenty of water. Whenever you feel slightly hungry, have a glass of water, and it will keep your hunger at bay. You should always carry a water bottle with you. Add in a couple of lemon slices, and mint leaves to make detox water.

Eat slowly

Whenever you eat, you should eat slowly. Don't be in a rush to stuff yourself. When you end your fast, you might feel the urge to binge on food. However, you should refrain from doing so.

Thoroughly chew your food before you swallow. And be sure and take small bites, cutting your food into bite-size bites the size that you would use to feed a child.

Eat healthy

You do want to lead a healthy life and lose weight, don't you? If yes, then you should be prudent about your diet. Be mindful of what you eat and don't binge on junk food. The food you consume during your eating window should provide your body with all the nourishment that it needs. After all, we are what we eat!

Cook at home

Try to cook at home as much as you can. If you don't buy prepackaged meals, you can considerably reduce your food bill. It might be easy to order a salad. However, it will prove to be expensive in the long run. Unlike the other fad diets, you don't need to buy any fancy ingredients. Cook at home and make sure that you eat what you cook at home. If not, it will only defeat the purpose.

Ration your portions

You should control the proportions of your meals. You can do this by simply measuring what you eat. Use weighing scales when you portion your meals. Your meals should be rich in protein and fiber while low in fats and carbs. Eat plenty of protein and fiber and your body will receive all the nutrients that it needs. Portion control is not a requirement, but can expedite weight lose.

Plan your meals

With intermittent fasting, you can choose your eating window. When you know your eating schedule, you can efficiently plan your meals. If you plan your meals, it will reduce the chances of wanting to eat out. If you know that you will fast the entire day, make sure that you have a meal waiting for you at home.

Grocery shopping

Whenever you decide to shop for groceries, make a list of all the ingredients you will need. Don't buy junk food. If you don't store any junk food at home, it becomes easier to eat a healthy diet. Out of sight, out of mind. So, keep your pantry stocked with healthy ingredients. Clean your cupboard of sugary carbs. Also, don't shop when you are hungry as it is quite likely that you will give into your urges to eat unhealthy foods. If you have all the ingredients you need to cook healthy meals, it is easier to cook. When you can plan and cook ahead, you can save yourself a lot of money.

Meal prep

You can do basic meal prep on the weekends and prepare for the week that lies ahead. Meal prep can be something as simple as cooking a stew and freezing it. Cut and portion the protein and vegetables you need. It helps reduce your cooking time, and you can whip up a healthy meal in no time. When you cook in batches, you tend to save money as well. Merely freeze whatever you cook and heat it up before you eat. You can even pack your meals and freeze them. Broth is one of the best things that you can cook in batches and freeze! You can use the broth to make soups, stews and curries.

Eat fruit for dessert

If you have a sweet tooth, it might feel challenging to give up on desserts. So, to satiate your sweet cravings, you can have fruit for dessert. A cup of strawberries with a tablespoon of unsweetened whipped cream is a tasty dessert. Have berries or any other fruit that you want. Fruit is good for your body and is full of nutrients. However, you should be mindful of the hidden calories. You shouldn't have two or three mangoes just because it is a fruit. For instance, frozen bananas with some peanut butter, or apple wedges with peanut butter make for a tasty sweet treat. There are plenty of healthy alternatives for desserts.

Food budget

You should set a weekly or a monthly food budget for yourself. When you plan your meals, you can efficiently allocate a weekly budget for yourself. It will help you to keep track of the expenses you incur on your groceries and other purchases.

Eat the healthy stuff first

When you break your fast, you will want to gorge on all sorts of foods. However, the idea is to eat healthy. So make sure that you eat all of the healthy foods before you think about eating anything that's not healthy. If you want a piece of chocolate or a scoop of ice cream, make sure that you fill yourself up with all the veggies and proteins that your body needs before you think about dessert. If you fill up on healthy foods first, you won't feel like you denied yourself a treat.

Brush your teeth after eating

It is a healthy habit to brush your teeth before you go to sleep at night. Make sure that you brush your teeth after dinner. In a way, it is a signal to your body that eating is over. It may seem small but it helps psychologically.

Don't leave the house hungry

How often do you buy coffee for yourself in the morning? Coffee might help to wake you up, but over time, the amount you spend on your morning fix-me up can be expensive. Why don't you make coffee at home and carry it with you? It is quite simple, and it will help you save money. Also, never leave home hungry. When you are hungry, you will feel like eating a lot of things that won't do your health or your bank balance any good. Instead, have a light snack before you leave.

Make your snacks

You don't have to buy diet snacks anymore. You can make your own 100-calorie snacks at home and carry them with you. You can whip up healthy, tasty, low calorie treats at home. For instance, you can make popcorn and store it up in small bags or containers. It can be your go-to snack. Similarly, kale chips are quite easy to make and are rather tasty. There are various options to choose from!

Track what you eat

You can maintain a food journal or use a food-tracking app to keep tabs on what you eat. The key is to make a list of everything that you eat. It will help you to eat healthy and cut down on mindless snacking.

Exercise

You don't need a gym membership to exercise. There are different ways in which you can exercise without going to the gym. Different no-cost exercise options include jogging, running, doing yoga at home, dancing and pure strength training exercises. Power up your laptop, pull up a few exercise videos, and exercise from the comfort of your living room!

We all have incredibly hectic schedules and lead busy lives and it can be difficult to follow a diet. However, you no longer have to worry about this. The tips in this chapter will help you to stick to your intermittent fasting diet, even if you have a hectic lifestyle. What's more? You can do this without burning a hole in your pocket.

Chapter Five:
Tips to Stay Motivated

Now that you know the different types of intermittent fasting and a whole host of tips that will help you lose weight, the next step is to start the diet. Have you ever tried a diet before? Do you feel that you tend to lose your mojo after a couple of weeks of dieting? If you want to obtain your health and weight loss goals, you should make sure that your motivation level stays high. Motivation will provide you the necessary strength to overcome any distractions and challenges that you might face. In this section, you'll discover simple tips to ensure that you don't lose motivation.

Set realistic goals

If you want to maintain your mojo when you start your diet, then you should set realistic goals for yourself. Before you think about cutting down a single calorie you should set the right target. In fact, your goals define your success in the long run. If you set unobtainable goals for yourself then you will set yourself up for disappointment. For instance, if you set an unrealistic goal like "I want to lose 30 pounds in three weeks" you will effectively set yourself up for failure. You wouldn't want that, would you? Set a goal that you can achieve. For instance, an achievable goal is "I want to lose at least one pound a week." The idea of intermittent fasting is to help create a sustainable and sensible pattern of eating that you can sustain in the long run. Set small and obtainable goals that you can accomplish that will help to motivate you.

Go slow

The success of a diet depends on the lifestyle changes that you decide to make. These changes take a while and they do not happen overnight. If you want to lose weight and make sure that it stays at bay, then you'll need to lose weight slowly. You can starve yourself and shed a few pounds, but it will not do you any good. The more gradual and steady your weight loss, the easier it is to maintain. Intermittent fasting is a great dieting option and it is sustainable. Make sure you go slowly. There is no hurry, and you don't need to jump right in.

Setbacks are common

Temptation can strike and there will be times when you might give in to your temptations. There is no harm in this, and once in a while, it is okay. The real trouble starts when you use a slip up as an excuse to binge. Call it the "I have already blown my diet, so I might as well eat a pint of ice cream." If you think like this, you will cause yourself a lot of unnecessary trouble. Treat a setback as an isolated incident and get back to your diet on the following day. After all, you are only human. It is okay to face a setback, but don't think of it as a failure. The attitude with which you deal with a setback can set the course for the rest of your diet.

Don't try to be a perfectionist

So, what would you do if you polished off a bag of Oreos? Perfectionist thinking gets in the way of success more than any other factor. If a 200-calorie indulgence is just that, "an indulgence" and nothing more, then it's okay. However, if you perceive it as a failure and a reason to give up, it can quickly turn into a 1000-calorie indulgence. Don't try to be a perfectionist when you start to diet. As mentioned in the previous tip, setbacks are expected and you should deal with them in a positive way.

Buddy up

Making a lifestyle change isn't all that easy and at times it might feel like an uphill battle. You aren't alone in this. You can find people who have similar goals to yours and buddy up with them. Different forums and groups help with dieting. Consider joining a group. If you don't want to do that, the next option is to find yourself a dieting partner. You can use your dieting partner for motivation, especially when you are running low on mojo. Your dieting partner can be your spouse, a family member, a friend, or even a colleague. Your buddy can keep track of your diet and exercise regime for you. When you are accountable to someone else, it improves the chances of your success.

Be patient

One of the significant obstacles to a diet is the weight loss plateau. You might eat right and exercise correctly, but the numbers on the scales don't seem to change. The scale appears to be stuck for some reason. Well, this is known as the weight-loss plateau, and it is something that every dieter faces. Merely turn around and congratulate yourself for your success so far. It is a part of the process of weight loss.

A simple trick that will help you to overcome this hurdle is to make slight changes to your diet. You can vary the macros you consume. Perhaps you can cut down on carbs and sugars and increase your protein intake. Or maybe you can double up on vegetables and cut out all fats from your diet. You can even try a different exercise routine to see if it changes things for you. Regardless of what you feel at that point, remember that this too shall pass. Be patient with yourself and don't give up on your diet. After all, you have made it so far and have successfully overcome all the other hurdles that stood in your way.

Reward yourself

Dieting does take some effort, and it might not seem fun at times. So don't forget to treat yourself when you achieve a goal. A goal could be big or a small. It could be something as simple as avoiding sugary treats for a day. When you achieve your goal, you should treat yourself. The reward doesn't have to be an extravagant one. Perhaps you can buy yourself a bottle of nail polish that you wanted! The rewards you set for yourself should never be food related. Don't reward yourself with a pint of ice cream for losing 5 pounds in ten days. It doesn't make any sense and renders the diet redundant. When you celebrate your success, it will make you feel better about yourself and your diet. Also, it will provide you with the necessary motivation to keep going even when you want to give up.

Maintenance plan

For a lot of people, losing weight seems to be easier than keeping it off. It is essential that healthy eating isn't a temporary change and it is a lifelong goal. It isn't a one-time project that you work on. You should design a maintenance plan for yourself so that you not only lose weight, but you can also make sure that you don't put it back on. The healthy habits that you develop on a diet will stay with you forever, and you shouldn't give up on them. If you want, you can always seek some professional help to come up with a maintenance plan.

Chapter Six:
Things to Expect

It is easy, once you get into the groove

It is easy to follow the diet once you get into your fasting groove. You can start your day with a cup of unsweetened tea or coffee. Then keep yourself busy with work until noon. At noon, you can have your first meal and make sure that you eat health. Your body is used to a specific diet or rather no diet up until now, and therefore it will take a while for you to get used to intermittent fasting. Fasting isn't that difficult, and it does get easier with time. Make sure that you keep yourself thoroughly engaged during the fast period. If you sit idly at home, then your mind will continuously think about food. The idea is to distract yourself from food. Concentrate on your work, indulge in one of your hobbies or do anything that you like. Create a schedule for yourself and stick to it. When you condition your body to eat at specific times and not all day long, it is easier to fast. Well, a good routine can't harm, can it? So, get started and create a schedule for yourself and plan your meals in such a manner that you won't feel too hungry when you fast. Also, include a little exercise!

Hunger Pangs

There is a lot of debate about breakfast being the most important meal of the day. The method of fasting that you opt for is entirely up to you. Hunger pangs are quite common during the initial week of fasting; don't get scared. Your body isn't used to fasting, and it will take a while to condition yourself to the diet. A hunger pang doesn't always indicate hunger. Confusing isn't it? At times, you will feel hungry when you are stressed or even bored. It is essential that you realize the difference between actual hunger and a natural craving. Ignore these pangs and get on with your day. Intermittent fasting doesn't mean that you should starve yourself, but at the same time, you shouldn't indulge in mindless eating either.

Benefits of exercise

When you exercise on an empty stomach you can burn more fat than you usually do. If weight loss is your primary goal, then you should try to exercise on an empty stomach. However, make sure that you don't take up any extreme forms of exercise. Even yoga on an empty stomach will increase your gains. When you exercise on an empty stomach, your body makes use of the stored fat to provide energy, and therefore it burns additional fat.

Change of perspective

Your perspective on food will change when you follow this diet. When you pay attention to what you eat and when you eat it, you will eat a whole lot healthier than ever before. The diet will make you conscious of the things you feed your system.

When you eat healthier, you will feel better, and your energy levels will increase.

The scale might not take a nosedive

During the initial couple of days of the fast, the scale might not make a nosedive. The weight you lose depends on several factors like your diet, metabolism, and age. You will lose some weight, but don't be disheartened if it isn't at the rate that you thought it would be. The weight loss is gradual, and you'll need to be patient. Patience and consistency are critical when it comes to Intermittent fasting. Don't give up on the diet just because you didn't drop thirty pounds in thirty days. Instead, give it some time, stick to the diet, and see for yourself. You cannot lose weight overnight. If you think you can, then you are merely setting yourself up for failure.

Now that you know what to expect on your new diet, you will be better prepared to manage it with success.

Chapter Seven:
When and What to Eat

In this section, you will learn about when and what to eat when you fast. If you know the answer to this, then you can make the most of intermittent fasting. There aren't any hard and fast rules about intermittent fasting, and one of the best features of this diet is the flexibility that it offers. You can eat the food that you like, and you won't feel that you are on a constant "diet." The phrase "food you like" doesn't refer to all sorts of unhealthy treats and you should show some prudence when it comes to what you eat.

When to eat on a fast day?

For a lot of people, fasting all day long and having a good meal in the evening is the best plan for a fast day. If your calorie allowance is around 500 calories on a fasting day, then you can have one meal that's worth 500 calories at the end of the day. You also have the option of having mini-meals all through the day as long as you stick to the calorie restriction. If you follow the crescendo method of fasting, then you will fast on two or three days of the week and eat like you usually would on all the other days. On the days that you fast, you can eat after your fasting window ends. It means that you can eat after you complete 12-16 hours of fasting. After you break your fast, you can have a light meal and follow it later with one or two meals. As mentioned, there are different forms of fasting that you can follow so select one that suits your needs. If you like to have a heavy dinner then you can save up your calories from the rest of the day and indulge yourself at night. A lot of people find it easier to wait until the evening to have a proper meal. If you fall into this category, then do so.

When you fast, you can have a couple of calorie-free snacks or maybe one low calorie bite, if you want. If you think you can do without the snack, then please do so! When you fast throughout the day, you might notice that your body is running low on fuel. In such a case, you can have a salty snack like a handful of popcorn! You can have a small bite during your fast, and it will not break your fast if you are careful about what you choose. Make sure that you drink plenty of water throughout the day. You can include a couple of cups of herbal tea or broth as well.

You'll need to remember that with intermittent fasting you can make your own rules. If you think you cannot fast all day long, you don't have to. You might like to have dinner and breakfast the following day, then you can. You don't have to worry about breaking any rules here. It is up to you and your comfort level.

What to eat on a fast day?

How can you make the most of your meals on a fast day? If all you can eat on a fast day is 500 calories, then make sure that you have as much protein and fiber as you can. If you follow a method of crescendo fasting or Leangains method, then make sure that you eat at least 1200 calories and don't go beyond 1500 calories. You can have two hearty meals within this calorie restraint. You shouldn't be afraid to fill yourself up with lean proteins like fish, eggs and chicken. You can even have lots of salad and vegetables. It is quite easy to fast once you get used to it.

Chapter Eight:
Frequency of Fasting

There are a lot of misconceptions that are associated with this diet, and in this section we'll bust the myths.

Skipping breakfast will make you gain weight

Breakfast might be considered to be the most important meal of the day, but it isn't, and that notion is nothing more than a myth. People believe that skipping breakfast leads to excessive hunger and weight gain. No scientific studies or research supports this claim. Skipping breakfast won't make you fat and you can do so quite safely without any fear.

Your metabolism improves when you eat frequently

It is a popular myth that eating frequently helps to improve your metabolism. Eating small meals does not improve your body's ability to burn calories. Yes, your body does need some energy to digest and assimilate the food you consume. It is referred to as the thermic effect of food, and it accounts for about 20-30% of total calories from protein, 5-10% from carbs and about 3% from fats. On an average, the thermic effect of food accounts for 10% of the total calories you consume. Take into consideration the total calories you consume and not the number of meals you eat. You don't have to keep eating regularly.

Eating frequently helps to keep hunger at bay

People believe that snacking continually helps to keep hunger at bay and reduces the chances of excessive hunger. Frequent meals will naturally leave you feeling full, but you don't have to do this. If you want to cut your cravings and keep hunger at bay, then you'll want to make sure that you are filling yourself up with the right kind of food. Your meals should contain high amounts of fiber, protein, and healthy fats instead of carbs. A meal that's rich in carbs will make you feel hungry soon and make you want to eat more food. Consuming carbs can make you crave more carbs. So, a balanced meal is the key to reducing your hunger.

Small meals assist in weight loss

Small meals won't do your body any good, and they certainly don't aid in weight loss. If you are worried that fasting leads to weight gain, you can lay those fears to rest.

The brain needs glucose

Yes, the brain needs glucose in order to function. It doesn't mean that you need to keep consuming carbs every couple of hours for your brain to continue working. It certainly won't stop performing if you don't eat anything for an extended period. This misconception is due to the assumption that the brain needs glucose for functioning. Your body starts producing glucose by a process known as gluconeogenesis. There is a reserve of glucose in the body, and your liver breaks this down to supply glucose that is essential for the functioning of your brain.

Eating often is necessary for proper health

Being in a fed state continuously isn't natural for the human body. During evolution, humans had to endure periods of starvation. If frequent meals were essential for survival, then the human race would have been wiped out a long time ago. In fact, fasting helps to induce cellular repair by kick starting the process of autophagy. It helps to protect against diseases like Alzheimer's and even certain types of cancers. Fasting is quite beneficial for the system, and it helps to cleanse the system by eliminating the build-up of toxins in the body. Snacking often has certain disadvantages. Frequent meals can easily increase your calorie intake and lead to a build-up of fatty cells in the liver.

Fasting shifts your body into "starvation mode."

A favorite argument against intermittent fasting is that it puts your body in starvation mode. While fasting, the body assumes that it's starving, and therefore shuts down its metabolism and prevents the burning of fat to produce energy. Long-term weight loss reduces the calories you burn, and that's what starvation mode is. However, this is bound to happen regardless of the dieting protocol you follow. Short-term fasting helps to speed up the metabolic function of the body. The increase in the levels of noradrenaline in the body increases the breaking down of the fat cells and thereby boosts the metabolism as well. Fasting for up to 48 hours helps to boost the metabolism, but anything more reverses this effect. You can fast as long as you follow a sensible fasting protocol.

You will lose muscle while fasting

Once again, it is nothing more than a misconception that fasting leads to muscle loss. Fasting leads to fat loss! In fact, intermittent fasting helps to increase the build-up of lean muscle and, when coupled with the right exercises, it helps to build muscle.

Chapter Nine:
Most Common Questions

What do I do about hunger pangs?

If you are someone who tends to eat every 2-3 hours, you might initially struggle a bit with controlling your hunger pangs, but it's not something that will build up to an extent that it will become unbearable. In fact, far from it! Here's what you can do when the cravings arise: you simply observe your body for about 30 minutes until it builds up, and then wait for another 15, and watch the hunger fade away on its own. Hunger pangs aren't something you can't cope with. It's basically your mind playing tricks on you, and although we agree that it's easier said than done, all you have to do is simply disconnect yourself from the feeling until it fades. If the hunger were so unbearable, our ancestors wouldn't have starved themselves until they could hunt their next meal. A lot of time we end up eating even when we are not hungry. Sometimes what seems like hunger could very well be that you are just thirsty and simply having a glass of water will suffice. Your body will remind you when you are actually hungry if you learn to watch how you feel rather than acting on your emotions. The feelings of hunger can be quite intense but don't last very long.

Can I drink alcohol during IF?

If your glass of alcohol contains less than 50 calories, then sure, go for it!! Let's be real here. A standard glass of wine can have anywhere between 120-155 calories depending upon what a standard glass is where you live. A glass of alcohol with as many calories as a mini-meal or a couple of snacks is certainly something you shouldn't be indulging into on your fasting days. Also, if you chose to drink a glass of wine instead of nutritional food, then your fasting days are going to be a real struggle. Beer is out of the question as it typically contains way more calories than wine. I don't want you to be hard on yourself but if you are into 5:2 IF, you can easily give up on the alcohol for those two fasting days rather than letting it sabotage the success this diet offers. You are fasting for a reason – to allow your body the rest it needs and let it detoxify and cleanse itself. If you are adamant about not giving up on your daily dose of alcohol during this span, you might as well not fast at all.

Won't IF slow down my metabolism?

All our lives we have been told that skipping our meals or spacing them too far apart will cause our metabolism to slow down. At the same time, the concept of eating smaller meals throughout the day was encouraged because of the belief that eating more frequently can accelerate your metabolism. So what's the real truth? If you drastically reduce your daily intake of food over an extended period of time, then chances are that your metabolism is going to slow down. Intermittent fasting does not involve any dramatic reduction in the calorie intake. If anything, it only compels you to eat healthier and more nutritious food while eliminating your snacking habits. Some studies show that intermittent fasting can, in fact, increase a person's metabolism, thereby resulting in weight loss. One reason is that having too much insulin in the body makes it a struggle to lose excess weight as it makes the body store fat. Intermittent fasting can lower your insulin levels to an extent that your body starts using fats as a primary source of energy, resulting in fat loss while increasing your muscle mass. You may be surprised to know this, but the amount of food you eat or the lack of it has nothing to do with your metabolic rate. In fact, your metabolism is closely linked with your body weight.

Won't I lose muscle if I'm not eating?

Almost all the studies conducted on intermittent fasting have been in regards to weight loss. It's important to know that without any physical activity, weight loss will naturally make you lose fat mass as well as muscle mass. The same applies for weight loss as a result of intermittent fasting as well as other diets. According to a few studies, some amount of lean mass (up to 2 pounds) may be lost after fasting for several months. But there are other studies that show no loss of lean mass even after fasting for longer duration. Some researchers also believe that in fact, fasting may be more useful to maintain lean mass during weight loss as compared to other diets. Overall, it is less likely that intermittent fasting will cause you to lose more muscle than other diets. It is a universal fact that when you lose weight, you tend to lose some lean mass as well as fat mass. This is especially true if you live a sedentary lifestyle and are not used to working out on a regular basis. So if you are keen on maintaining or gaining more lean muscle mass, you will have to perform regular weight training exercises while following this diet.

Why is this diet better than other diets?

If you have been looking for strong reasons that assure your intermittent fasting is actually better than other diets, we may just have to explain it to you in detail. Here are the reasons:

It helps you lose weight and your nasty sugar cravings

Ever felt like you can't live without that chocolate cake? Chances are that it's the very reason behind your love handles. As per studies, people who have successfully managed to burn more fat due to intermittent fasting have also found that their sugar cravings disappeared.

It builds muscle and helps to maintain overall health

Intermittent fasting is not just a diet; it's a way of life. So you can expect excellent health without sacrificing your muscle mass. This is one reason why most athletes seriously consider adding intermittent fasting to their daily regime.

It improves brain health and protects you from Alzheimer's

A study conducted by the National Institute of Aging shows that fasting every other day can spike up the brain-derived neurotrophic factor. BDNF is basically a brain-boosting protein that encourages neural health and improves your brain health as well as protects you from Alzheimer's.

It reduces stress and prevents cancer

Intermittent fasting enhances insulin sensitivity and mitochondrial energy efficiency, which helps to slow down the aging process of your body. Intermittent fasting is also associated with cancer prevention and treatment because cancer cells are unable to use fat as fuel and they require sugar to thrive.

Will I lose weight and fat?

Yes. Let me explain how. The primary reason intermittent fasting has proven to be highly effective in weight loss is because you end up consuming fewer calories. All the protocols surrounding intermittent fasting suggest skipping meals for longer durations. This means you are ingesting fewer calories unless of course, you end up overeating during the eating window. Although weight loss isn't only measured by your calorie intake, it can certainly be mediated by an overall decrease in calorie consumption. There have been several studies conducted on intermittent fasting that have shown that people are able to lose more weight per week as they continue fasting. Some people have also reportedly lost up to 7% of waist circumference, implying that it has also helped them lose belly fat.

Fasting forces your body to use the stored fat as a source of energy. When you burn calories this way, rather than through eating food throughout the day, it helps to lose weight as well as the excess fat storage in your body. Intermittent fasting optimizes the release of vital fat burning hormones in the body. This includes insulin as well as Human Growth Hormone (HGH). HGH plays a significant role in triggering the body's fat burning furnace.

What should I eat after my intermittent fast?

One of the most important aspects of learning how to carry out intermittent fasting is to know how to ease back into your daily diet. The first thing you need to do after finishing your fast is to forget that you ever fasted. Yes, I said that! Pretend the fast never happened.   This also means no reward, no compensation, no binges and no specific way of eating. Just get back to your regular diet without changing anything. The moment your fast comes to a halt, simply erase it from your memory and eat just the way you have been eating. If you end your fast during lunchtime, eat lunch. If the fast ends at 5:00 PM and you generally don't eat your dinner until 7 or 8 pm, feel free to eat a light snack (keep it below 50 calories) but ensure that you don't eat anything substantial until it is mealtime.

There is no secret way or time to end your fast. And there's no magic wand that can make you forget that you ever fasted. Once you end the fast, give yourself a few minutes and think about your daily meal times and carry on as if you never fasted. It's not as difficult as you think. Once you start training your mind to ease back into your daily meals as soon as the fast is over, you will find the whole process easier. What generally happens with most people who take up intermittent fasting is that they tend to start craving healthier foods towards the end of their fast. Instead of digging into a tub of fries or a slice of pizza, they end up drinking a healthy smoothie or eating fruit. If you are someone who gets similar cravings, don't hesitate to consume something healthier at the end of the fast.

Can I exercise when fasting?

That's a big YES! There's absolutely no reason why you shouldn't be exercising when intermittent fasting. We would encourage you to try as many different forms of exercise as possible. You need to try out different exercises every week, not only to keep boredom at bay but also to keep yourself motivated. If you are not big on exercise and have been a couch potato all your life, don't jump your guns and take up intense exercises like mountain biking or running. Take up a light activity like walking or yoga and then slowly increase the intensity of your workouts.

A lot of people avoid working out during fasting due to the fear of losing muscle mass. As long as you are training two or three times a week then you won't lose any muscle. In fact, intermittent fasting can actually boost your growth hormones, thereby preventing muscle loss. You may notice that your energy levels might go down a bit if you perform high-intensity work out on the day you are fasting, but it shouldn't be a point of concern. However, you may experience fatigue sooner than on a typical eating day. If you feel slightly more exhausted than usual, just end your fast a bit earlier.

As per studies, exercising on an empty stomach can have a number of health benefits. When you combine fasting and exercise, it optimizes the impact of catalysts and cellular factors that accelerate the breakdown of glycogen and fat for energy. This, in turn, forces the body to burn fat and spike up your metabolism.

Will I get a headache from not eating? If so, can it be prevented?

No, not always! Not everyone gets headaches while doing intermittent fasting. Now there has been a lot of research carried out on fasting and headaches. These results show that women are more prone to headaches during fasting. Many assume that this happens due to dehydration, but that's not the case. These headaches are similar to the withdrawal symptoms you experience once you quit an addiction – for instance, quitting coffee, smoking or drinking.

Reasons why you get headaches during fasting include:

- You might get a headache because your blood pressure levels are either too high or too low.

- A decrease in sugar levels in your body can cause a headache during fasting.

- People who gulp down several cups of coffee during fasting are bound to feel dehydrated by the end of the day, thereby triggering headaches.

- If you are anemic, chances are high that you will experience headaches during fasting.

- Lastly, people with sinus issues are likely to develop a headache while fasting.

From my personal experience, if you experience headaches during fasting, they go away after the first two or three days. It will take your body time to adjust to a new routine. You can treat your headaches with over the counter medications or home remedies, just like you normally would when you are not fasting.

Additional Tips:

Don't eat too much food when you break your fast. Overeating during meal times redirects more blood flow to your stomach, resulting in a terrible headache.

If you already have a headache before you break your fast, try chewing on dates. Dates are extremely light on the stomach and contain a balanced amount of sugar required by your body to regain strength.

Ensure you are properly hydrated during your fast. Drinking plenty of water before and after your fast is important to keep you from dehydration. Avoid caffeinated drinks and soda, as they could be the reason why you end up dehydrated the day after the fast.

An important tip that can soothe your headaches in minutes is to soak your feet in warm water, keep something cold behind your head and lie down for a while.

I was told if I don't eat every three hours I could faint because my blood sugar level will drop. How do I prevent this?

Our society is somehow convinced that hypoglycemia, lightheadedness, shaking and fainting will occur if we skip a meal or two or even if we exercise in a fasted state. But have you ever considered the possibility that the perceived symptoms of hypoglycemia could be because of anxiety and not because of skipping meals? It's a known fact that perfectly healthy people do not experience a drastic drop in their blood sugar levels while fasting. In fact, even a 24 hours fast will not make you vulnerable to hypoglycemia.

As long as you are healthy, your blood pressure isn't going to swing from one extreme to another. So, no, you won't feel weak, faint or experience lightheadedness if you skip a couple of meals. Your body's internal mechanism is capable enough to maintain your blood sugar levels even when you aren't eating. You may assume that you can't nail intermittent fasting because you may have the habit of eating from morning until you go to bed. It's natural for you to assume that skipping your meals will make you hungry.

Let me explain in detail why eating every three hours is the very reason you could feel hungry all the time. Your body is being supplied with a steady stream of carbohydrates that is suppressing the body's endogenous glucose gland production. Your body does not need to tap into the stored fats or glycogen for energy, but it is your habit of constantly stuffing yourself with food that is making you hungry. Fasting can actually help in this case as it has a suppressive effect on hunger. Always remember, there is enough glycogen storage in the liver to fulfill your body's immediate energy requirements. And when your body burns that stored glycogen through fasting, you won't feel dizzy or pass out, as your body will eventually break down fat for fuel.

Will this fast work for me?

I get it. You are plagued with doubts right now because chances are that you are trying hard to lose weight and don't know which diet you should choose. To be honest, there is one common problem with weight loss and the pursuit of general well-being and wealth. A lot of people say they wish to "try it out," but they aren't nearly as committed as they claim.

What are the most popular ways of doing the intermittent diet?

One of the top favorite approaches to intermittent fasting is the "eating window" approach. This technique consists of 4-10 hours window, and the only time you can eat is during the remaining 14-20 hours. Although this method is simple, some people can find it quite difficult to follow, especially during the initial few days. The designated eating window ensures that your fast is followed religiously, but the strictness of this technique can discourage a lot of dieters from taking it up. That being said, a lot of people who are desperately trying to lose weight swear by this method. Once your body adapts to this kind of fasting method, you probably won't find it too hard to stick to.

Another favorite technique among the dieters is, "The Warrior Diet." Most people experience positive results within weeks of following this technique. The Warrior Diet, created by the famous, Ori Hofmekler, requires you to eat only tiny portions of snacks consisting of fruit, nuts, and veggies during the day while compensating the calories during the last meal of the day. While The Warrior Diet is not considered as a fast, following this protocol does offer great psychological benefits and allows you to consume larger meals, even at a calorie deficit. These are some of the reasons why people love this type of fasting.

Who should and shouldn't do intermittent fasting?

Most people can follow this type of fast without experiencing any side effects. However, there are certain groups of individuals who shouldn't fast. Take a look below:

Teenagers

When we are still growing we need enough food every day. If you are under 20, fasting could mean eating fewer calories than what your body requires, and that's not good for your overall health.

Pregnant women

For obvious reasons, women who are pregnant need to eat sufficient food, as they are eating for two. Pregnant women should not try out any type of diet, let alone intermittent fasting, without consulting with doctor.

People with type 2 diabetes or hypoglycemia

Several researches claim intermittent fasting can actually help to treat and potentially eliminate Type 2 diabetes. However, this is very speculative, and there hasn't been strong evidence supporting this claim. What we can assure you about fasting is that it can certainly help you control your blood sugar levels if you take insulin, thereby alleviating the symptoms. Intermittent fasting does not trigger it, but if you are already suffering from it, you should only try fasting while under close medical supervision.

People who are anemic or who have an eating disorder

Fasting helps your body burn fats. But if you are anemic, you certainly don't have enough fat storage in the body to burn and use it as a source of energy, and you will end up burning more muscle instead. This could be life threatening for someone who is suffering from anemia. Similarly, if you suffer from an eating disorder you are going to face the similar issues.

Other health problems

It's always a smart move to get a physical before you decide to make dietary changes. This will help you identify underlying medical conditions, if any, and you can be sure to follow an appropriate health plan. It's also important to have your blood sugar levels, weight, and cholesterol levels checked before you start fasting. Then, check once again within a span of month or two and track the progress. This could be a great way to keep yourself motivated and help you stick to the plan.

What about Children and elderly?

The safest diet for a child is no diet, just healthy eating. Avoiding junk food and sodas from an early age will help a child get a great head start on self care. However, the elderly can absolutely give it a try unless they are suffering from a severe medical condition that restricts them from dieting. The elderly can benefit from the life-extending, neurological and health-promoting advantages of fasting. It can help slow the progression of certain age-related ailments, enhance the quality of his or her life and improve overall health, leaving them feeling energetic and positive.

I socialize and eat out a lot, how am I going to cope with it?

First of all, know that you can have cheat days. Cheat days can help you prevent the feeling of losing out on your favorite food. There's some scientific evidence that cheat days accelerate our metabolism. So there's no need to feel deprived! We quit most diets because they are difficult to follow, especially the ones that don't mesh with our lifestyle. If you have ever followed a crash diet or the so-called "quick fix diet," you know how much of a struggle it can be. On the other hand, intermittent fasting isn't as restrictive as it seems. You can certainly continue socializing and still follow the fast. Intermittent fasting does not require you to give up certain foods or insist that you turn into a vegan, go wheat-free, or eat clean.

Also, your friends and family may surprise you by supporting your new eating habits. For all you know, there's someone out there waiting to be inspired so they can join you for the fasting. After all, everyone's looking to bring positive changes to their dietary habits these days. There are so many people out there who wish to take up intermittent fasting but lack the drive to do so, and you can end up being his or her inspiration. So eating per your diet or eating at parties or any social situations shouldn't be hard. If you have to go out for a late dinner, post your eating time, eat something light (typically a snack less than 50-60 calories). There's absolutely no reason why you should give up on your fasting protocols just because you like socializing.

How much weight am I going to lose?

Although people generally end up losing a good amount of weight when they take up intermittent fasting, that shouldn't be your main goal. And if you are really big on losing weight, you may have to try different intermittent fasting diets to see what works best for you. And even after that, needless to say, how much weight you lose completely depends upon your body. Typically, you can expect to lose anywhere between 1-1.5 pound in a week. Most people who have gone through complete transformation say that sometimes the weight loss isn't immediate and it took a few weeks before they started shedding the extra pounds. Your body needs adjusting, so allow it some time to find its balance. Once it adapts to the new diet, you will start losing weight easily. Just don't expect dramatic results immediately. It could be that you may consistently lose weight over a period of weeks, months or even a year. The key is to be patient with yourself and your body. You might want to try another diet if you are looking to lose 10 pounds in a week. But I'm betting that the weight will be back on, and you will slip into your old eating habits within a short time.

What if I am in perfect shape and don't want to lose any weight while fasting?

That's great! If only more people were as content as you. Here's the thing: there are people who don't wish to lose any weight and still benefit from intermittent fasting. Contrary to the popular belief, weight loss isn't the only thing that this type of fasting offers. As per studies, people tend to perform their worst post eating hours. We all wake up with a list of things we want to finish within the day, but as soon as the sun goes down, we experience a sudden drop in energy. Haven't you been in a situation where you thought you could work on a presentation post dinner, but instead hit the sack as you eat? Plus, nighttime is when most people tend to drink. Chances are that you like to have a glass of wine to de-stress at night. The point I am trying to make is that nighttime is the most vulnerable. It's when people often tend to make bad choices. When you are fasting, you automatically get into the habit of not rushing towards your temptations, and that means you will easily avoid junk and sugary items. Even if you don't wish to lose weight, I am sure you are interested to keep your body fit, am I right? If you are in search of a good diet, fasting can certainly do you some good. It's more than likely that you are eating something far less good for you, and that is what's making you want to follow a diet plan. Well, if that's the case, you should totally try fasting.

How long can I safely fast?

As per clinical studies, water fasts that last for 24 to 36 hours are well tolerated by the body and are generally considered safe. From a maintenance and weight loss perspective, water fasting for 24 hours on a regular basis can be extremely difficult to follow and would not be recommended as a healthy practice. On the other hand, alternate day fasting with regards to food is known to benefit a large chunk of people. Individuals who follow these fasts have reported to experience a dramatic decrease in their depression as well as binge eating habits. It has also helped people get over body image issues and maintain a positive outlook towards their body.

In order to keep your metabolic health intact, it's advisable to stick to a fasting regime that suits your lifestyle. In short, don't be too hard on yourself. If alternate day fasting or 5:2 fasting seems easier, go for it. In case you experience discomfort or feel light-headed, immediately see your physician. Intermittent fasting is pretty safe as long as you don't pick a drastic method of fasting or you have underlying medical issues that can make it harder to fast.

I can go without food for the entire week, but I am worried that I won't be able to stick to it during weekends, is that okay?

Yes! This, in fact, is a good way to train your body to adapt to any dietary changes. Rather than fasting all seven days and then eventually getting exhausted with such a strict regime, it's always better to do the 5:2 intermittent fasting. In this method, you fast five days a week and eat normally for the next two days. Just because you can't fast on Saturdays and Sundays, it doesn't mean that you can't do it during the weekdays. Giving yourself a rest for two days does not nullify the advantages you get from following it for the other five days.

You should be applying the same principle to everything else you do. This goes for weightlifting, swimming, running or even cycling. Is eating a single healthy meal in a day better than not having anything healthy at all? Absolutely. Is squatting once a week better than not squatting at all? Exactly! Remember, that just because you can't do something perfectly well doesn't mean you should completely abandon it.

Is there anything I can eat between fasts or will that defeat the purpose?

This is a great question as it can clear up a lot of misconceptions about intermittent fasting. Let's start with the basics. You can certainly eat whatever you want during the eating period. You can look at it as fasting as well as a feeding window. That said, don't go eating like there's no tomorrow. The key is to not overeat. Listen to your body, and notice how you feel after you eat a certain portion of food. If you feel close to full, stop eating. Although you are not restricted to two or three meals a day and are free to eat whatever you want, ensure that you don't overeat.

In the fasted state, you ideally cannot eat anything. If you are not used to fasting and are struggling to keep up with it, try eating a small fruit or anything that has less than 50 calories. The reason behind taking up intermittent fasting is that you want to allow your body to rest and go without having to continuously digest food. If you keep snacking in between, there's really no point to follow this fast. And yes, that will certainly defeat the purpose.

Conclusion

All the information that you need to follow an intermittent fasting plan is provided in this book. You can choose from any of the different variations of the diet until you find one that works well for you. Intermittent fasting is more of a change in your lifestyle rather than just a diet. If you want sustainable weight loss and want to lose fat along with it, then you should stick to this diet. You can see positive changes in your body within a month of following this diet.

Please keep in mind that the concept of intermittent fasting stresses when you can eat instead of what you can eat. However, it doesn't mean that you stuff yourself with unhealthy junk food and then complain that there isn't any weight loss. Show some prudence when you eat, include a little exercise, and you can turn your health around.

Intermittent Fasting is not only beneficial to your health, but it is also easy to follow. A few lifestyle changes and you can reap the benefits that this diet has to offer.

Well, all that's left now is for you to get started.

We wish you the best of luck.

Recommended Reading

SUGAR: Shut Your Mouth To Sugar Addiction And Cravings Forever

http://bit.ly/sugarhog

AUTOIMMUNE DISEASE ANTI-INFLAMMATORY DIET

smarturl.it/autoa

DUKAN DIET: Four Phase Plan To Lose Weight FAST And FOREVER

http://bit.ly/dukandietsa

References

https://caloriebee.com/diets/How-to-Lose-Weight-and-Eat-Healthy-on-a-Budget

http://paleoforwomen.com/shattering-the-myth-of-fasting-for-women-a-review-of-female-specific-responses-to-fasting-in-the-literature/#

https://blog.kettleandfire.com/intermittent-fasting-for-women/

https://www.precisionnutrition.com/intermittent-fasting-women

http://journals.plos.org/plosone/article?id=10.1371/journal.pone.0052416